LOCALIZED FAT:

Is it possible to eliminate localized fat?

TABLE OF CONTENTS

INTRODUCTION

I want to thank you and congratulate you for downloading the book Localized fat: Is it possible to eliminate localized fat?

This book contains proven steps and strategies on how to lose weight

Here's an inescapable fact: Many of us can be stubborn, frustrated, and reluctant to strive to seek out the good form and improve the look of our body. But we know how and why people fail these programs and all the mistakes they make along the way, plus how to prevent that from happening.

CHAPTER 1

Why can't I lose weight?

If you always wonder why you can't maintain a diet or exercise program, here's what might be your problem.

You're not plotting realistic goals

Biting more than you can chew is the biggest recipe for failure. In the world of weight loss, the biggest mistake is to be unreal with yourself. Most people prepare for failure by setting unreachable goals.

This is especially true if you have no previous experience! Someone who eats junk and doesn't train, does all the wrong things, and suddenly in a week decides to start exercising, eating healthy and doing all those things he didn't do, always ends up frustrated and without progress.

You want instant results

If you have already done a workout and wondered why you do not have a flat belly afterwards, you are not alone. We are in this world of instant results, where everyone wants something from day to night!

Don't expect to lose weight faster than you've gain before. Imagine that you have gain 25 pounds in the last five years, but after a week of training, you already think: "I did everything" and already gets frustrated.

It was only a week. You gain 25 pounds in a week? Then don't expect the opposite to happen.

You're not being honest with yourself. Be honest and work with reality. If you haven't been to the gym for a decade, you won't train every day from now on unless you're hyper-motivated and have a superhuman determination.

You need to choose the steps, plan and specific tools you can accomplish reasonably. Don't follow any plan just because someone you know has succeeded in that.

You're making excuses

The biggest problem is the apology. Everyone has an excuse. It could be your thyroid, or the busy day. But everyone has time to watch Netflix, but no one has time to exercise.

When you inspirational stories like that, you realize there's no excuses. If you really want something, you go get it.

The solution

"Limit yourself" is probably not the weight loss advice you expected, but it makes sense. Set realistic goals. Set one or two small goals per week, like eating a healthy breakfast every day and drinking more water.

Once you feel that you have mastered this small task (which may be more difficult than you think), only then should you start addressing more responsibilities.

You can establish training twice a week for a month. After this month, try training three times a week... progresses in smaller steps. Get rid of the excuses and get ready for success. That's how you stop yourself from failing in the journey for weight loss.

CHAPTER 2

What is the best diet to lose weight?

Diet to lose belly: Herbal foods can accelerate fat burning and help in that goal.

Losing belly is the desire of many people, and feeding is usually directly related to the localized fat in this region. Most of the time, this accumulation of fat comes from the ingestion of simple carbohydrates, present in breads, pasta, sweets, soft drinks and alcoholic beverages.

Besides the aesthetic discomfort, the belly is usually a risk factor for cardiovascular health. Cholesterol, hypertension, diabetes and other health problems may arise when the waist is higher than indicated.

If losing belly is on your list of goals, some foods can accelerate fat burning and help in that goal.

What to eat in the diet to lose belly

1. Fish and Seafood

Inflammation is one of the main responsible for weight gain. Fish and seafood, because they are rich in omega 3, an essential fatty acid, help to unignited fat cells, acting in control of the problem and helping to lose belly. In addition, these foods also accelerate the transformation of glucose into energy, preventing it from being stocked in the form of fat. The inclusion of these foods on the menu can be done at least three times a week.

2. Safflower oil and other functional oils

Functional Oils Act on fat metabolism, increasing the breakdown of fatty acids for energy production and, consequently, decreasing fat reserves. Safflower oil and coconut oil also act in the acceleration of metabolism.

3. Yoghurt with Probiotics

Some lactobacilli produce a type of fat, the CLA (conjugated linoleic acid), which is able to reduce the percentage of fat. In addition, this type of food has the basic function of balancing the intestinal flora. A study published in 2006 by the scientific Nature journal showed that bacteria present in the intestinal flora of people with obesity are very different from those of people with adequate weight. The discovery suggests that inadequate absorption of fats in the intestine, which occurs in people with compromised flora, may be related to weight gain.

Probiotics also benefit the functioning of the intestine, reducing stomach stuffing related to gases and intestine trapped. Some examples of food with probiotics are yoghurt with lactobacilli.

4. Integrals

The integrals are rich in fibers, which are important allied in the process of losing belly. The first reason is that consuming fibers with plenty of water helps improve intestinal transit, which prevents the belly from being stuff and swollen. In addition, fiber-rich foods tend to have a lower glycemic index. This is because the fibers decelerate the glucose absorption of the foods, avoiding spikes in glycemia and the hormone insulin, responsible for bringing the sugar to the cells. Carbohydrates with lower glycemic index are: Sweet potato, brown rice and chia.

5. Red Fruits

The red-purplied berries (raspberry, blackberry, strawberry, cherry, blueberry, watermelon and purple grape) are powerful allied to lose belly. There are, in the shells of these fruits, phytochemical substances with antioxidant action, such as Anthocyanin, which maintains the circulatory system efficiently, improving the irrigation of tissues and helping in the burning of abdominal fat. It is recommended to consume one or two cups a day, without adding sugar.

6. Green Tea

In addition to acting in the central nervous system, accelerating metabolism and increasing body temperature, xanthines (caffeine, theophylline and theobromine) present in coffee, green tea, black tea, matte tea and chocolate increase the mobilization of stored fats, helping to lose belly. You can take a cup of tea from 30 to 40 minutes after lunch and dinner, with special care not to consume it before sleeping (which may disrupt sleep) and if you are hypertensive, because these substances increase blood pressure.

7. Hibiscus Tea

A research published in the Journal of Ethnopharmacology of the International Society of Ethno has concluded that Hibiscus tea is able to reduce adipogenesis, process in which cells mature and become able to accumulate fat, i.e. it is an excellent ally to lose belly. It is still unclear what is the substance present in the beverage that is responsible for the benefit. However, it is believed that the antioxidant action of the flavonoids anthocyanin and quercetin contributes to reduce the fat deposition.

8. Ginger

Ginger is a thermogenic food, which helps accelerate metabolism and increase fat burning, being an excellent support for losing belly. Gingerol, the main compound, exerts antioxidant, antifungal, anti-inflammatory functions, inhibits platelet aggregation, avoiding the appearance of Thrombi. The indicated amount of ginger is two small slices per day. That's enough to have the thermogenic effect.

9. Olive oil

A survey conducted by the Instituto Salud Carlos III, from Spain, in partnership with the University of

Cambridge, of England, points out that daily intake of olive oil avoids the formation of fats in the waist region. The study was published in the journal Diabetes Care and states that the monounsaturated fats present in the olive oil prevent the accumulation of fat in the region.

Olive oil is an excellent food to prevent cardiovascular diseases, since it has anti-inflammatory components that act in the vessels, decreasing the aggregation of fat.

10. water

All reactions of our organism depend on water. To burn fat, eliminate toxins, intestine work properly and avoid fluid retention we need to drink water.

What not to do in the diet to lose belly

Sleep little: During sleep our organism produces leptin, a hormone capable of controlling the sensation of satiety throughout the day. Therefore, people who have difficulty sleeping produce smaller amounts of leptin. The consequence of this is exaggerated intake of calories during the day, because the body does not feel satisfied

Taking a soda: feeding with more caloric beverages only increases the danger of increasing weight and ingest liquids that contain gas, such as soft drinks, causes the stomach to dilate and impair the absorption of nutrients. The person feels falsely satiated, returns to hunger shortly afterwards and, worse, ends up extrapolating the consumption of food in the next meal

Fast eating: The sensation of satiety, that is, that we are satisfied, is sent by the brain to our body approximately 20 minutes after we start eating. Who eats fast, ends up consuming more than it should, because it does not give adequate time for the perception of satiety by the brain.

Spend a lot of time without eating: diets that involve spending long periods of fasting are harmful to the organism. The orientation is to eat from 3 in 3 hours, and the period without feeding should not exceed a maximum of 4 hours.

CHAPTER 3

How to lose weight fast?

Slimming: 20 tips to lose weight fast and with health. Follow the tips to boost your diet and eliminate your tummy.

To lose weight with health it is necessary that the body spends more calories than it consumes. That's why the two most important measures to reach the ideal weight are adjusting eating habits and practicing physical activities. But this should be done gradually and with a healthy and varied menu. Follow the tips for healthy weight loss:

Consume foods that burn fat

Some foods help to lose weight because they stimulate fat burning. The hibiscus tea, Lyia, cranberry flour are among them.

Consume foods that Deswell

Foods Rich in Omega 3 (salmon, tuna, sardines, herring, mackerel, flaxseed, chestnuts) contribute to the slimming due to anti-inflammatory action. Meet the anti-inflammatory diet.

Increase satiety

Foods rich in fibers provide greater satiety, so hunger takes longer to appear, which helps you to lose weight. The main sources of fibre are: fruits, whole grains such as rice, wheat, rye, barley and oats. Vegetables, such as beans, lentils, chickpeas and peas, and vegetables and vegetables also have good amounts of fibers. The seeds, such as chia, flaxseed and pumpkin seed, also have fibers.

Consume foods that accelerate metabolism

Foods with thermogenic action stimulate greater calorie burning. The main thermogenic foods are: pepper, green tea, cinnamon, ginger and coffee.

Make snacks

The ideal when you want to lose weight is to make the three main meals (breakfast, lunch and dinner) and two or three small snacks. This will keep your metabolism running all day long, give you more satiety, lessening hunger out of time, and prevent you from exaggerating in big meals. The interval between each meal must be at least 2 hours.

Invest in a balanced and varied dish

A healthy diet demands balance of nutrients and variety of foods. It is worth investing in fruits, vegetables. Do not forget to complete the menu with different types of meats, cereals, beans, lentils, milk and derivatives, food groups essential for daily feeding.

Avoid making restrictive diets

Diets that drastically cut calories or some specific component, such as carbohydrates for example, are considered restrictive. To lose weight with health the expected is to lose between a pound and a kilo per week. More of this may be a sign that you are not performing the most appropriate diet. The monotonous feeding and with little variety of food does not bring all the nutrients that the body needs, and may even affect the immunity and the body more vulnerable to diseases. Diet of shakes, gluten-free diet and soup diet are some examples of restrictive diets.

Invest in teas that help you lose weight

Some of them, such as green tea, black tea and cinnamon tea, stimulate caloric burning. While Hibiscus tea contributes to less fat being accumulated in the abdomen.

Practice fat-burning exercises

The World Health Organization recommends practicing at least 150 minutes of moderate exercises per week for a person to be considered active. That is, practicing 1 hours of exercise in three days in the week (180 minutes), you already exceed this goal! To burn fat and lose weight it is important to invest in aerobic activities such as: hiking, jogging, biking, dancing, and swimming, among others.

Be sure to gain muscle

Practicing strength exercises, such as bodybuilding and Pilates, are also super important to gain muscle and make the body spend calories.

Be careful with the fashion diets

There are a number of diets that promise rapid weight loss. Stay tuned to what cost this weight loss is achieved. Many of them lead to loss of muscles, which is especially harmful for those who want to lose weight and keep their weights after that. Some of these diets are:

Reduce salt and sugar consumption

Salt is the main source of sodium, which in excess mineral in the body increases the risk of hypertension and fluid retention. Sugar consumed in excess is transformed into fat accumulation, mainly in the belly region. Food sources of simple carbohydrates are rich in sugar. Among them are: addition sugar, soft drinks, sweets and those with lots of white flour, such as breads, pasta and cakes.

Know when something is wrong with the diet

Some signs that rapid weight loss is damaging your health are: hair loss, weak and brittle nails, discouragement, weakness, indisposition, dizziness, sagging, and intestinal constipation.

Stay away from trans fat

This type of fat can be found in some biscuits, ice creams, industrialized cakes, among other foods. Trans fat increases LDL (bad cholesterol for the body) and decreases HDL (good cholesterol). In addition, it also acts by increasing the triglycerides that can be stored in the adipose tissue.

Reduce saturated fat consumption

The consumption of excess saturated fats is related to the accumulation of fat in the body, that is, difficulty to lose weight. Foods with large amounts of saturated fats are: red meats, whole milk, butter and cheeses.

Drink an average of 2 liters of water per day

Consuming the right liquids contributes and

greatly to weight-loss in a healthy way. The recommendation is to ingest between 30 to 35 ml per kg body weight of liquids, which on average is around 2 liters per day.

Find out what your ideal weight is

Body mass index (BMI) is a way to assess whether the person's weight is within the considered healthy or not. It is calculated by weight in kilograms divided by the squared height (kg/m²). Although it does not show the proportion of fats and muscles of the human body, the BMI helps to have a notion about whether the weight of the individual is within the considered healthy or not.

Reduce daily calorie consumption

For fast weight loss many people opt for an extreme reduction of calories. Consumption less than 1200 calories per day is not oriented to weight loss and can lead to problems such as weakness, fainting and, of course, accordion effect.

CHAPTER 4

When a person greatly slimes what can be?

Low weight: Know when slimming can be dangerous.

The scales are always popular, especially for women. The war is to make you point numbers inferior to the ones you see. But in a few moments, the scale can show these numbers smaller than expected, announcing that something may not be right with the organism.

A body below the ideal weight can conceal health problems such as diabetes and hyperthyroidism, among other evils, as well as may cause disturbances that even reach life at risk. Knowing the causes and consequences of low weight is essential for the maintenance of health and well-being.

It's not what it looks like

It is common sense to observe a person who is underweight and to associate his thinness with malnutrition. However, not all the squalid are necessarily suffering from the lack of nutrients. It is necessary to take into account the individual characteristics of each, in addition to calculating Body mass index (BMI), because there are those who present low weight and high percentage of fat in their bodies and vice versa. The BMI is very important, but we have to have good sense and evaluate the biotype of each person. There are women, for example, with a stronger structure, which will cause them to be heavier and, not so, are above the ideal weight.

Malnutrition is usually caused by a diet that is low in calories and proteins, or by poor absorption of nutrients. It may be the summation of several causes, such as social, psychiatric or pathological. Therefore, every person who is out of the ideal weight, both for more and less, should seek a skilled professional to rule out a more serious condition.

Free-Fall Hands

Sudden weight loss should always be investigated. After all, diseases such as hyperthyroidism, some types of cancer, type I diabetes, hepatitis C, bulimia and anorexia can lead to abrupt loss of the pounds not always desired. Staying with a slender body is cool, but health should not be compromised, because these illnesses are serious and can even lead to death.

Everyone wants a perfect body, but some people don't know how to achieve it in a healthy way. This is because weight loss can also be induced through restrictive diets, which end up compromising health. Some of the consequences that this sudden slimming brings to the body are amenorrhea (absence of menstruation), hormonal imbalance, weakening of the nail and hair, changes in mood and sleep, change in skin color, fall of immunity, among other. The low weight is dangerous by itself, but in women, for example, it can seriously compromise fertility, because sex hormones are derived from fat, cholesterol.

Age also ends up influencing weight loss. The gynecologist of the pregnant clinic recalled that, with the advancement of the years, it becomes more difficult to lose weight spontaneously, which makes the attentions double in case of severe slimming. On the other hand, self-image disturbances, such as anorexia and bulimia, tend to affect younger individuals. In these cases, the extreme weight loss leads to the risk of death due to failure in the functioning of some organs, since their needs are not supplied.

Counting on fingers

To find out if you have the ideal weight, you need to prepare to calculate the BMI, stipulated by the World Health Organization (WHO). This number takes into account the height and weight of the person, in a generalized way, to determine whether the individual is obese, in the ideal or overweight. The Formula is the division of his body weight by height, elevated squared, in meters.

So, pencil and paper in hand (or Calculator): Formula: weight (kg) / [height (m)]2. The result shows how the relationship with the balance goes.

-below 16: malnutrition;

-Between 16.1 and 18.4: below weight;

-Between 18.5 and 24.9: normal weight;

-Between 25 and 29.9: overweight;

-Over 30: obesity.

It's back

When losing too much weight in a short period of time, it is necessary to investigate the cause of the slimming. The best way is to seek a physician to perform examinations that will point out the cause of the low weight. It is also interesting to seek a nutritionist for a food reeducation aimed at increasing body mass. In the case of eating disorders, such as bulimia and anorexia, therapeutic accompaniment is still indicated.

Stress and anxiety can also affect weight loss, being indicators that the body needs to Step on the brake. For these cases, complementary therapies such as acupuncture, florals, phytotherapy, chromotherapy, Holistic massage, among others, to help remedy the problem.

CHAPTER 5

How to lose the belly Fat?

How to slim your belly fast – 10 tips.

If you have a type of fat that seems to be the most stubborn in your body, it's probably abdominal fat. Depending on your genetics, you may have propensity to gain weight in the abdomen or not. Some people gain weight mainly in the abdomen, while mainly women see the size of their thighs and buttocks increase. You will be able to understand how to reduce your belly quickly if you first understand why it is there – and why the diet is more important than workouts.

Having abdominal fat can disrupt your life in many ways. Not only does it make you wear certain types of clothes, but it also makes you look older and affect your posture. If you're tired of dealing with your abdominal fat, here are some great tips on how to reduce your tummy fast.

1. Take care what you eat

If you want a miraculous cure or a quick way to lose your tummy and not get it back, it's time to come to reality. The only true way to avoid abdominal fat is to have a healthy diet. It's that simple. If you eat more calories than burns, you gain weight. Thus, you can begin to notice your abdomen increasing when you increase the consumption of highly caloric foods and beverages such as fast food, unhealthy foods and alcohol.

If you really want a high-strung belly, you need to take care of your diet. You don't have to count your calories, but you should focus on eating raw foods with simple ingredients. Fruits, vegetables, whole grains, lean meats and low-fat dairy products should be the most part of what you consume. If you focus on eating good food and limiting enough unhealthy foods, your abdominal fat will disappear and will not come back.

2. Keep an eye on food calories

Cutting the amount of calories you consume is the first thing you need to do if you want to get rid of your abdominal fat. Once you reduce the amount of calories you consume, your body will compensate you for it by burning the fat stored in your body naturally. However, do not assume that having a calorie-free diet is the answer to your abdominal fat problem. The right amount of calories is essential to the functioning of your body and your health, so always consult an expert before deciding to make any drastic changes in your diet.

Looking at the food label is a good way to control calorie consumption. Be aware that carbohydrates have 4 calories per gram, while proteins also have 4 calories per gram and fats have 9 calories in each gram. Learn how to decipher food labels.

3. Decrease alcohol

Alcohol is a toxic substance to the body and the liver gives preference to metabolize it first. This change in liver metabolism favors the accumulation of fat in the body

If you like to party on the weekend or sit down with a beer or two after a day's work, one of the ways you can lower your calorie intake is to avoid beer. The beer contains many calories. In addition, alcoholic beverages also cause inflammation in your organs. To stay safe, avoid caloric beverages completely, such as soft drinks and energy.

4. Decrease sugar

In addition to calories, sugar is an important contributor in the formation of abdominal fat. The sugar that is found in soft drinks, sweets and other unhealthy foods burns very fast in body, so if you consume these foods without exercising afterwards, the sugar will become fat automatically and be stored in the body. Of course, sugar is also found in healthy foods like fruits and some vegetables. However, the sugars from these sources take longer to burn.

5. Avoid evening snacks

Another effective tip for you to know how to slim your tummy is to eat early. Don't eat long before you sleep because snacks at night are not burnt before you sleep. Instead of being used as energy, the most calories just add more fat to your abdomen. If you feel the need to eat or drink something before bedtime, try an herbal tea or a small amount of skimmed milk.

6. Eat smaller portions

Decrease your food intake if you are overweight or obese. Eating smaller portions of healthy foods is an effective way to lessen your belly fast.

7. Start walking

Many people seek how to slim the belly without any exercise, but the truth is that no matter how hard you try, you will not be able to lower your abdomen if you do not do any kind of exercise. If you don't like intense workouts, you can just start walking more. Walking is probably one of the easiest exercises you can do, and it is also one of the most effective. If you don't work away from your house, leave the car and walk. The same thing is worth if you go to the grocery store or do something else. Not only will you get rid of your abdominal fat, but you will also do a favor to the environment.

8. Exercise regularly to burn calories

Aerobic exercises burn calories that increase the size of your tummy. The more calories you burn and the fewer calories you consume, the lower your abdomen will be. Cardio exercises of 40 minutes three times a week will help you lose weight and get in shape. Pilates exercises are especially beneficial for sculpting and tonifying your whole body, including the abdomen. You can take Pilates classes at most gyms.

9. You cannot lose localized shape fat

Don't be fooled by expensive abdominal device commercials that promise you a flat abdomen in a few weeks. Exercising is important in any plan for health and wellbeing, but caring for what you eat is much more important to lose and maintain weight. You should also note that it is impossible to aim for a specific area of your body to lose weight. Doing 200 crunches a day won't give you a flat abdomen. Even if you eat healthily and exercise beyond the ABS or other exercises focused on the abdomen. In the end, it's your genetics that decides.

Exercising is the most effective way when combined with a healthy diet. The abdominal fat will not stay away just with the exercises. You should focus on most of your efforts to eat well and add exercises as a secondary measure.

10. Be patient

There is no miracle cure or quick fix. Adopting a healthy lifestyle is the only way to have a flat belly. Don't expect the fat to disappear in just a few weeks. Give your body time to adjust to healthy habits. That kind of change doesn't happen overnight!

In short, you have to be willing to make lifestyle changes to know how to slim your belly fast. However, just follow these tips correctly.

CHAPTER 6

The diet of the boiled egg to lose weight

There are few diets that promise a rapid and miraculous weight loss. It has one that restricts carbohydrates, another that only allows proteins, and even one that only allows fruit. What almost all of them have in common is that they are highly restrictive and fail to promote food reeducation.

By eliminating an entire food group (as is the case with the fat-free diets, or the low carb diets, which practically prohibit the consumption of foods rich in carbohydrates), these diets can cause nutritional deficiencies and inevitably end up taking to the unwanted accordion effect. In other words, many of these miraculous diets even lose weight, but the probability of getting fat again is quite high, since there was no alteration in eating habits, but only the exclusion of certain foods.

In this scenario, the cooked egg diet seems to be a

slightly more reasonable option, since it does not exclude any food groups or suggests a very low calorie intake. It is important to understand how the diet of the cooked egg to lose weight, the menu and tips to not re-fatting again with the accordion effect.

What is the boiled egg diet?

This diet consists of consuming a poached egg or cooked before the three main meals daily – breakfast, lunch and dinner. The diet bias of the boiled egg to lose weight is to increase satiety with the egg and reduce calorie consumption during the next meal.

All of this, of course, in conjunction with a slightly hypocaloric diet – that is, it contains fewer calories than its metabolism needs to perform its daily activities. This means that the cooked egg diet is a calorie-restricted food plan that utilizes the highest satiety power of proteins to cause a weight loss without you needing to starve as in other highly restrictive diets.

How does the diet of the boiled egg to lose weight?

Why include three eggs in the diet? Does the egg lose

weight? There are, in fact, several reasons why consuming boiled eggs before the meal can be a good idea for those who are trying to lose weight.

See why:

1. The egg brings satiety

The egg is rich in proteins and fats – are about 6g each per unit – two nutrients that have digestion slower than carbohydrates and therefore bring more satiety. To be broken into amino acids, egg proteins require great energy expenditure on the part of the organism, which is obliged to withdraw energy from its reserves to aid digestion.

That is, consuming a food rich in proteins and without carbohydrates as the egg accelerates the metabolism and causes a mobilization of the fat stocks – especially the abdominal, leading to an increase in lipolysis (fat burning) to aid in digestion. Therefore, we can say that the boiled egg burns fats (in the absence of carbohydrates).

Consuming an entire egg before each meal will make you feel satiated with a smaller amount of food in the next meal, facilitating the maintenance of the Hypocaloric diet.

And that statement has scientific proof. In a

study conducted by the Rochester Center in the United States, researchers found that egg consumption at breakfast can decrease calorie consumption throughout the day – can be up to 400 calories less in a period of 24 hours.

In the study, 30 overweight or obese women received a breakfast containing either two eggs or a bagel (a type of ring-shaped bread) with an add-on, and the two options had the same amount of calories and proteins.

After accompanying the eating habits of the study participants throughout the day, the researchers were able to notice that those who had consumed the eggs at breakfast felt less hungry before lunch, and as a result ended up consuming fewer calories during the meal. And it wasn't just that: during the next 36 hours, the group that ate eggs consumed, on average, 417 calories less than the one who received the bagel at the first meal of the day.

It is worth remembering that, in order for you to get a similar result, your diet should be hypocaloric.

2. The egg is source of vitamin B12

Vitamin B12 helps you to lose weight in an indirect way. This is because it helps to metabolized proteins and fats, producing energy that makes the organism more active during the day. This means that vitamin B12 stimulates metabolism and can aid in reducing body fat reserves.

In addition, vitamin B12 present in the egg will leave you with more energy and willingness to exercise, which can also help in weight loss.

3. The egg is a source of tryptophan

The egg is one of the best sources of tryptophan, an amino acid that stimulates the production of serotonin (a type of neurotransmitter) in the brain. Among other functions, serotonin can control appetite and decrease food compulsion, as well as decrease anxiety and stress.

Adequate levels of tryptophan in the body can decrease the will to eat sweets and facilitate the process of slimming through a decrease in hedonic hunger – that is, that hunger that appears even when the body is not with energy deficiency.

4. Eating eggs does not cause glucose spikes

This is a very interesting egg property, especially in the morning. As we wake up, our glucose is down there (after all, we stay at least 8 hours fasting) and all our bodies need is a carbohydrate source to restore their normal blood sugar rates.

It turns out that if you consume a carbohydrate soon when you wake up and without a protein source together, your glucose levels go up there very quickly, which obliges the body to release a large amount of insulin to throw that glucose inside of the cells. And guess what happens when all the glucose goes into the cells? That's right, your sugar levels go down again, in what's known as the famous glucose spike.

When that happens, your brain sends a signal to feed you again, which means feeling hungry right after you've just eaten a slice of bread and jelly. And the bad news is that this occurs throughout the day as well, because when we stay without feeding for many hours the glucose rates fall dramatically.

As it has slow digestion and does not contain carbohydrates, the egg does not cause large fluctuations in blood glucose, which will help you control your appetite in the first meal of the day. Consuming an egg before the main meal can help you stabilize your glucose without having to suffer sudden changes in appetite immediately afterwards.

5. Eggs favor the synthesis of adiponectin

The consumption of eggs can increase the production of adiponectin, a hormone that accelerates metabolism, increases fat burning, improves insulin sensitivity and decreases appetite.

But the egg doesn't increase the cholesterol?

The egg is without a shadow of doubts the most controversial food in our food; in a day is the best food in the world, in the other one should not even look at it. Fortunately, however, much of the research carried out in recent years has not only acquitted the egg as it even recommended its consumption. So it seems a good idea to adopt the diet of the boiled egg to lose weight.

For a good portion of medical professionals, the consumption of up to 3 eggs during the week does not increase cholesterol and can still be beneficial to health. This is because, as we have already seen, the egg is the source of a series of important nutrients for health, being considered one of the most complete foods in the world.

In addition, scientists have proven that cholesterol consumption in the diet does not necessarily increase cholesterol levels in blood circulation. The justification would be that the liver already produces a large amount of cholesterol every day. Thus, when we consume eggs in the diet, the liver tends to produce less cholesterol, keeping the rates of total cholesterol in circulation stable.

Research suggests that, for 70% of the individuals, the egg has no effect on cholesterol, while for the remaining 30% the consumption of eggs can slightly elevate the rates of LDL (bad cholesterol).

Some people, however, have familial hypercholesterolemia, an inherited condition that is characterized by high rates of LDL in the blood, regardless of the consumption of cholesterol in the diet. For those who present the condition, the consumption of eggs (the clear ones are usually allowed) should be avoided, at the risk of raising even more the rates of total cholesterol.

Try to eat the egg without salt, as the sodium increases the retention of liquids and will leave you swollen;

Do not fry or add fat to the eggs. To increase satiety, the egg must be cooked and, at most, accompanied by a natural seasoning, such as oregano or parsley;

An egg contains approximately 70 calories, which will give a total of 180 calories (for three eggs) to be included in its daily sum;

Do not diet for more than a week, since the amount of eggs is very large and can cause problems to the kidneys;

Continuing with your normal feeding and simply

adding an egg will not make you lose weight; On the contrary, you may even get fat if you choose to simply add three eggs to the diet without making changes in eating habits;

Drink plenty of water, both to facilitate the elimination of toxins and decrease the swelling as to protect the kidneys, which may be overloaded by processing the large amount of protein from the eggs;

Do not make this diet if you have a history of kidney problems or elevated levels of LDL (bad cholesterol);

Resist temptation and make no omelette, scrambled egg or fried egg. Limit yourself to the boiled egg, to prolong digestion and increase satiety without exaggerating the calories;

Lastly, remember that there is no miraculous diet, and only food reeducation and daily practice of physical activity can make significant and permanent alterations in their weight.

CONCLUSION

Thank you again for downloading this book!

I hope this book was able to help you to understand the important of food reeducation.

The next step is to practice daily physical activity.

Finally, if you enjoyed this book, please take the time to share your thoughts and post a review on Amazon. It'd be greatly appreciated!

Thank you and good luck!

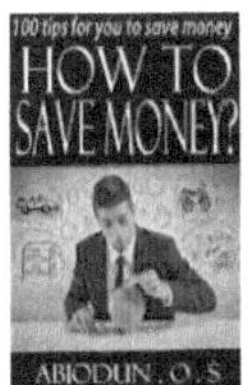

How To Save Money:Money Management, Budgeting, Kindle Short Reads, Self-Help, Books, Business and Money, Personal Finance, Budgeting & Money Management: 100 tips for you to save money Mar 25, 2016

by Abiodun Oluwasegun S , Abiodun Oluwasegun. S

Kindle Edition

$4.98 $4.98

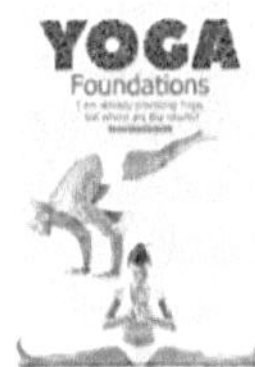

YOGA Foundations: I am already practicing Yoga, but where are the results? Dec 29, 2018

by SHARAFA ABIODUN

Kindle Edition

$6.66 $6.66

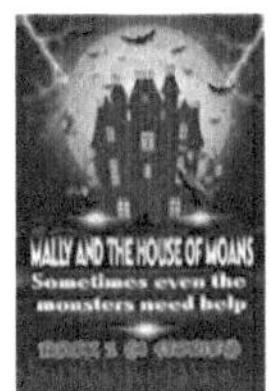

SHARAFA ABIODUN

Kid's book:"MALLY AND THE HOUSE OF MOANS": Short spooky stories for kids (monster, monsters, monster books for kids, kids books and kids book): Sometimes ... Short spooky stories for kids Book 1) Jan 1, 2016

by Abiodun Oluwasegun S

Kindle Edition

$5.49 $5 49

(20)

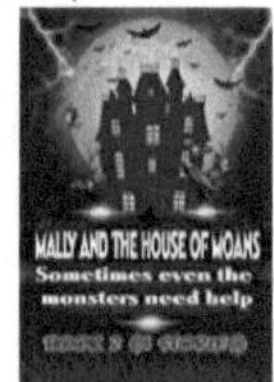

Kid's book:"MALLY AND THE HOUSE OF MOANS": Short spooky stories for kids (monster, monsters, monster books for kids, kids books and kids book): Sometimes ... Short spooky stories for kids Book 2): Kid Jan 15, 2016

by Abiodun Oluwasegun S

Kindle Edition

$5.54 $5 54

(1)

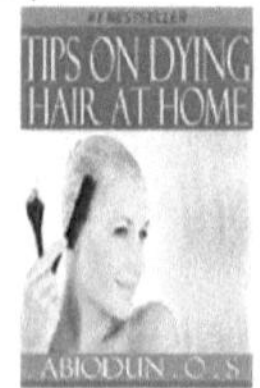

Tips On Dying Hair at Home: Dye Hair, Crafts, Hobbies & Home, Fashion, Hair, Dye, Beauty, Grooming, & Style, Self-Help, Health,

Fitness & Dieting (Tips ... & Style, Self-Help, Health, Book 1) Mar 26, 2016

by Abiodun S

Kindle Edition

$0.97 $0⁹⁷

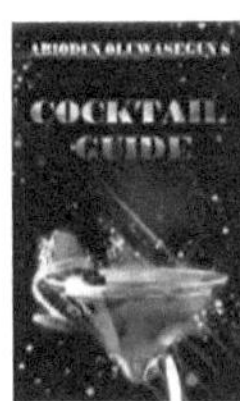

Cocktail guide:cocktail guide, Bar Book, Cocktails, Amazon, Books Feb 14, 2016

by Abiodun S

Kindle Edition

$3.17 $3¹⁷

Paperback

$15.00 $15⁰⁰

Get it by Friday, Feb 01

(2)

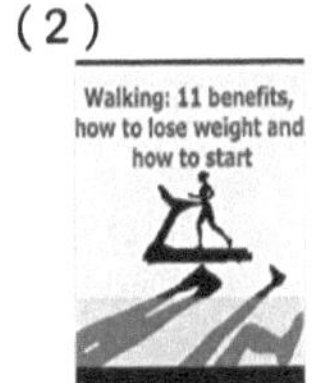

SHARAFA ABIODUN

Walking: 11 benefits, how to lose weight and how to start (3 Book 1) Jan 25, 2019

by SHARAFA ABIODUN

Kindle Edition

$6.63 $6 63

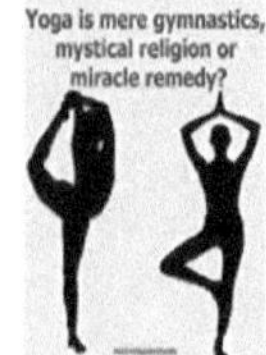

Yoga is mere gymnastics, mystical religion or miracle remedy? Jan 18, 2019

by SHARAFA ABIODUN

Kindle Edition

$6.65 $6 65

Paperback

$10.00 $10 00

Get it by Friday, Feb 01
More Buying Choices
$9.99 (3 Used & New offers)

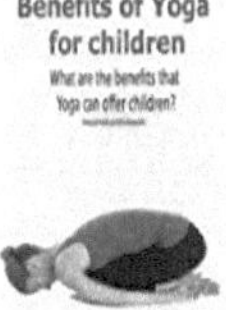

Benefits of Yoga for children: What are the benefits that Yoga can offer children? Jan 3, 2019

by SHARAFA ABIODUN

Kindle Edition

$6.73 $6 73

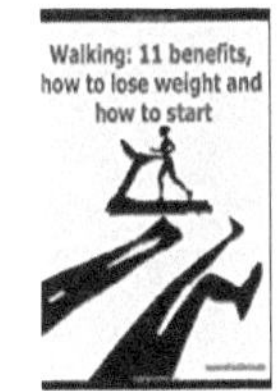

Walking: 11 benefits, how to lose weight and how to start (3) Jan 26, 2019

by SHARAFA ABIODUN

Paperback

$10.00 $10 00

Get it by Friday, Feb 01
More Buying Choices
$10.00 (3 Used & New offers)

SHARAFA ABIODUN

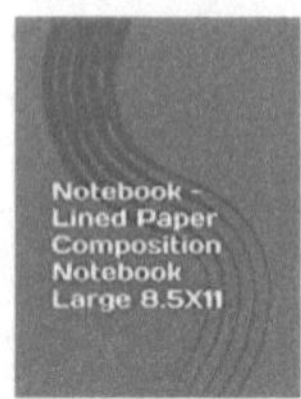

Notebook - Lined Paper Composition Notebook [Large 8.5X11] Jan 5, 2019

by SHARAFA OLUWASEGUN ABIODUN

Paperback

$10.00$10.00

Get it by Friday, Feb 01
More Buying Choices
$10.00 (4 Used & New offers)

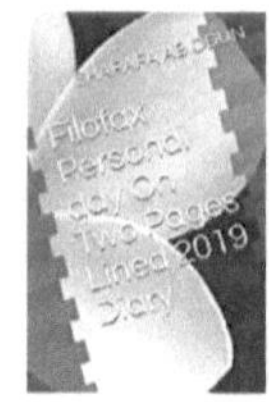

Filofax Personal day On Two Pages Lined 2019 Diary- Diary Jan 3, 2019

by SHARAFA OLUWASEGUN ABIODUN

Paperback

$15.00$15.00

Get it by Friday, Feb 01

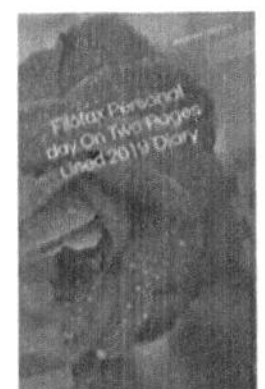

Filofax Personal day On Two Pages Lined 2019 Diary Jan 2, 2019

by SHARAFA OLUWASEGUN ABIODUN

Paperback

$15.00 $15 00

Get it by Tuesday, Feb 05
More Buying Choices
$14.54 (5 Used & New offers)

2017 Daily Dashboard - Journal, Diary, Notebook: Journal, Diary, Notebook (Volume 1) Feb 5, 2017

by Abiodun Oluwasegun. S

Paperback

Out of Print--Limited Availability.

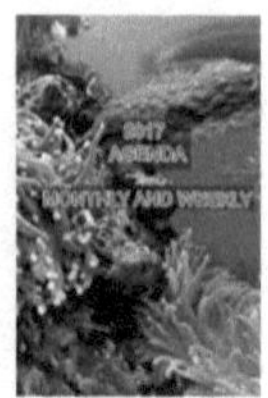

2017 Agenda: Monthly And Weekly (Volume 1) Feb 4, 2017

by Abiodun Oluwasegun. S

Paperback

Out of Print--Limited Availability.